WEIGHT LOSS SMOOTHIES

30 Delicious and Nourishing Smoothies for Weight Loss and Good Health

Sarah B. Smith

Table of Contents

Introduction

"Unlock the Secret to Vibrant Health and Sustainable Weight Loss with 30 Irresistible Smoothie Creations. Welcome to a journey that combines the delight of flavors with the science of nutrition. In this book, you'll discover a collection of carefully crafted smoothie recipes that not only tantalize your taste buds but also pave the way for your weight loss goals. Each sip is a step towards a healthier you, as we blend the finest ingredients to create a symphony of flavors that nourish, energize, and help you shed those extra pounds. Get ready to embrace a lifestyle where health and indulgence harmoniously unite, sip by sip."

Chapter One: An Overview

A smoothie: a sumptuous concoction of blended whole food(fruits, vegetables, yogurt, or other ingredients) artfully crafted to harmonize flavors, textures, and nutrition, resulting in a refreshing and wholesome elixir that invigorates the senses and fuels the body's vitality.

While the concept of the modern smoothie might not have existed for ages, the consumption of blended beverages made from various ingredients has been a part of many cultures throughout history. Traditional societies often combined fruits, vegetables, herbs, and even dairy products to create concoctions that offered several potential benefits:

Nutrient Intake

Blending ingredients can make it easier to consume a variety of nutrients in a single serving. Ancient civilizations recognized the value of combining different foods for better overall nourishment.

Digestibility

Blending breaks down food into smaller particles, potentially aiding in digestion and making nutrients more accessible to the body. Historical societies may have used this method to enhance nutrient absorption.

Hydration

Many traditional beverages were based on blending water with fruits or other ingredients, offering hydration along with vitamins and minerals.

Preservation

Blending and fermenting ingredients were methods used to preserve foods before modern refrigeration. Fermented beverages like kefir or kvass have beneficial probiotics, which are now linked to gut health.

Medicinal Value

Certain blended mixtures in various cultures were used as tonics or remedies for specific health concerns. For example, Ayurvedic practices include blended herbal concoctions for healing.

Elderly and Infants

Blended foods were often suitable for those who had difficulty chewing, such as the elderly or infants transitioning to solid foods.

Culinary Creativity

Blending allowed for creativity in combining flavors and ingredients, leading to the development of regional specialties.

Cultural Practices

Different cultures had their variations of blended beverages that held cultural and ritualistic significance.
Just some few benefits to whet your appetite, now let's dive into the delicious recipes that revitalize the body, mind, and soul!

Chapter 2: Health Benefits of Smoothies

How smoothies alone can improve your health in the best ways possible

Smoothies are a nutritional powerhouse that can significantly elevate our health. Packed with vitamins, minerals, fiber, and antioxidants, they offer a convenient way to consume a variety of nutrients in one delicious drink. Incorporating smoothies into our diet can enhance digestion, boost energy levels, and support weight management. By blending whole fruits, vegetables, and even protein sources like Greek yogurt or plant-based protein powder, we can easily meet our daily nutrient requirements.

Smoothies also promote hydration, which is essential for optimal bodily functions. They can be tailored to specific health goals, such as improving immunity, promoting skin health, or aiding post-workout recovery. Their high fiber content aids in satiety and can help control hunger, potentially leading to better portion control and weight maintenance. Additionally, smoothies can be enriched with ingredients like flaxseeds, chia seeds, or spinach, further enhancing their nutritional value.

However, it's important to balance smoothie ingredients to avoid excessive sugar or calorie intake. Incorporating a variety of ingredients ensures a diverse nutrient intake. While smoothies can offer substantial health benefits, they should be part of a well-rounded diet that includes whole foods from different food groups.

Why smoothies will melt away fat

Smoothies can be a valuable addition to a weight loss journey due to their nutritional composition and potential to aid in fat loss. Packed with essential vitamins, minerals, and fiber, they offer a convenient way to consume a variety of nutrients. By including ingredients like leafy greens, fruits, and protein sources such as yogurt or plant-based protein powder, smoothies can help keep you satisfied while promoting satiety and reducing cravings.

The combination of nutrients in smoothies can support metabolism and energy expenditure, which are key factors in fat loss. Ingredients like berries and citrus fruits provide antioxidants that can aid in reducing inflammation, potentially contributing to improved metabolic function. Additionally, the fiber content in smoothies can slow down digestion, leading to better blood sugar control and reduced hunger.

While smoothies can be beneficial, it's important to maintain a balanced diet and consider portion control. Using whole, nutrient-dense ingredients and avoiding excessive added sugars or calorie-dense additives is crucial. Regular exercise and overall healthy lifestyle choices complement the effects of smoothies in achieving sustainable fat loss. Remember that no single food or beverage can magically "melt away" fat; it's the combination of smart food choices, physical activity, and consistency that ultimately contributes to weight management and overall well-being.

How smoothies will jumpstart your weight loss

Smoothies can serve as a positive catalyst for jumpstarting your weight loss journey in a natural and wholesome manner. By carefully selecting nutrient-rich ingredients, these beverages offer a convenient and satisfying way to support your goals. Incorporating a balanced blend of fruits, vegetables, lean proteins, and healthy fats can provide essential vitamins, minerals, and fiber that enhance metabolism and curb appetite.

The hydration aspect of smoothies also plays a role, aiding digestion and promoting a feeling of fullness. Starting your day with a well-portioned smoothie can set a nourishing tone and encourage mindful eating throughout the day. Moreover, the versatility of smoothies allows for creative combinations that cater to your personal preferences and dietary needs.

Incorporating whole foods into your smoothies, such as leafy greens, berries, and nuts, ensures that you're benefiting from their natural goodness. While smoothies can kickstart your weight loss, they work best when integrated into a comprehensive lifestyle approach that includes regular physical activity and balanced meals. Remember, the journey to weight loss is a gradual process that requires patience and consistency. Smoothies can be a supportive tool, but the overall commitment to a healthy lifestyle is what truly propels sustainable weight loss.

How to boost your smoothies to make them healthier

Smoothies are a convenient and tasty way to pack nutrients into your diet. To boost their health benefits, consider these tips. Start with a nutrient-rich base, like a mix of leafy greens and low-sugar fruits. Adding protein, such as Greek yogurt, nut butter, or protein powder, helps with satiety and muscle repair. Incorporating healthy fats from sources like avocados, chia seeds, or flaxseed can enhance nutrient absorption and provide sustained energy.

Including fiber-rich ingredients like oats or psyllium husk promotes digestion and helps maintain blood sugar levels. Consider adding superfoods like spirulina, acai, or matcha for an extra antioxidant boost. Enhance the flavor and nutrients by using unsweetened almond milk, coconut water, or even green tea as a liquid base.

Avoid excessive added sugars by skipping sugary juices or sweetened yogurt. Instead, opt for natural sweetness from ripe fruits. Add spices like cinnamon or turmeric for their anti-inflammatory properties and unique flavors. Lastly, balance is key – be mindful of portion sizes and the overall calorie content, especially if weight management is a goal.

Remember, variety is essential to ensure you're getting a wide range of nutrients. Experiment with different ingredients and ratios to find the combinations that best suit your taste preferences and health goals.

Chapter 3: Ingredients used in smoothies and their flavor profiles

Let's start with some popular fruits, vegetables, superfoods, proteins, and other ingredients used in smoothies, along with their nutritional benefits and flavor profiles:

Fruits:

Bananas:
Creamy texture and natural sweetness. High in potassium, vitamin B6, and dietary fiber.

Berries (Strawberries, Blueberries, Raspberries, Blackberries)
Bursting with antioxidants and vitamins. They add a tangy-sweet flavor.

Mango

Tropical sweetness with a hint of tartness. Rich in vitamin C and vitamin A.

Pineapple
  Refreshing and slightly tangy. Contains bromelain, an enzyme that aids digestion.

Kiwi
  Tangy and slightly sweet. Excellent source of vitamin C, vitamin K, and dietary fiber.

Vegetables:

Spinach
The mild flavor blends well. Packed with iron, calcium, and vitamins A and K.

Kale
Earthy and slightly bitter. High in vitamins C and K, as well as antioxidants.

Cucumber
Refreshing and mild. Adds hydration and a crisp texture.

Carrots
 Sweet and slightly earthy. Rich in beta-carotene and vitamin A.

Avocado
Creamy and rich texture. Offers healthy fats, potassium, and fiber.

Superfoods:

Chia Seeds
 The gel-like texture when soaked. High in omega-3 fatty acids, fiber, and antioxidants.

Flax Seeds
A nutty flavor with a crunch. Rich in omega-3 fatty acids and fiber.

Spirulina
Blue-green algae with a strong flavor. Contains protein, iron, and various vitamins.

Matcha
Green tea powder with an earthy taste. Provides antioxidants and a gentle caffeine boost.

Acai Berry
Dark purple fruit with a berry-cocoa flavor. Loaded with antioxidants and healthy fats.

Proteins:

Greek Yogurt
Creamy and tangy. Packed with protein, probiotics, and calcium.

Plant-Based Protein Powder
Comes in various flavors. Suitable for vegans and those looking to increase protein intake.

Nut Butter (Almond, Peanut, Cashew)
Creamy and nutty. Offers protein, healthy fats, and vitamins.

Silken Tofu
Smooth texture with a neutral taste. Contains plant-based protein and is low in calories.

Other Ingredients:

Coconut Water
  Hydrating and slightly sweet. Contains electrolytes and potassium.

Oats

Adds thickness and fiber. Provides sustained energy and promotes digestion.

Honey or Maple Syrup
Natural sweeteners. Use in moderation for added sweetness.

Ginger
Spicy and warming. Aids digestion and adds a unique flavor.

Remember, the combinations of these ingredients can create a wide range of flavor profiles and nutritional benefits. Feel free to experiment and find your favorite combinations!

Chapter 4: Tips and Techniques

Smoothie Tips and Techniques

Discover the art of crafting nutritious and delicious smoothies with these expert tips and techniques. From selecting fresh, vibrant fruits and vegetables to incorporating protein-rich ingredients like Greek yogurt or plant-based protein powders, this guide will show you how to create a symphony of flavors that nourish your body. Learn the secrets of balancing sweetness with greens, experimenting with superfoods, and achieving that velvety smooth texture for a delightful and healthful smoothie experience.

Here are some basic tips for making a great smoothie:

1. **Ingredient Ratios**: Aim for a balanced combination of fruits, vegetables, protein, and healthy fats. A common ratio is 2 parts

fruits/vegetables, 1 part liquid, and 1 part protein/fats.

2. **Liquid Choices**: Choose a liquid base such as water, milk (dairy or plant-based), yogurt, or coconut water. The amount of liquid can vary based on how thick you want your smoothie.

3. **Fruits and Vegetables**: Use a variety of fresh or frozen fruits and vegetables. Common choices include bananas, berries, spinach, kale, and mango. Frozen fruits can make your smoothie thicker and colder.

4. **Protein and Fats**: Add a source of protein (e.g., Greek yogurt, protein powder, nut butter) and healthy fats (e.g., avocado, chia seeds, flaxseeds) to help keep you full and satisfied.

5. **Sweeteners**: Opt for natural sweeteners like honey, maple syrup, or dates if needed. Be mindful of the sweetness of fruits.

6. **Extras**: Consider adding extras like oats, nuts, seeds, or spices (e.g., cinnamon, ginger) for added flavor and nutrition.

7. **Blending** Techniques: Start by adding the liquid and softer ingredients first. Then add the frozen or harder ingredients on top. Blend on low to break down large pieces, and gradually increase to high for a smooth consistency.

8. **Texture Control**: Adjust the amount of liquid to control the thickness of your smoothie. If it's too thick, add more liquid; if too thin, add more fruits or ice.

9. **Prep Ahead**: Pre-cut and freeze fruits and vegetables to save time. You can also

prepare smoothie packs with measured ingredients for quick blending.

10. **Experiment**: Don't be afraid to experiment with different ingredient combinations to find your favorite flavors and textures.

Remember, there are no strict rules—customize your smoothie to your taste and nutritional preferences!

Chapter 5: Smoothie Recipes

Recipe 1

Green Protein Power Smoothie

Ingredients

- 1 cup spinach (fresh or frozen)
- 1/2 cup kale (fresh or frozen)
- 1/2 banana
- 1/2 cup mixed berries (blueberries, strawberries, raspberries)
- 1/2 cup low-fat Greek yogurt
- 1/2 cup unsweetened almond milk (or any milk of your choice)
- 1 tablespoon chia seeds
- 1 scoop of your preferred plant-based protein powder (optional)
- Ice cubes

Nutritional Values (approx.)

- Calories: ~250
- Protein: ~15g
- Fiber: ~8g
- Healthy fats: ~8g
- Carbohydrates: ~35g

Preparation

1. Add the spinach, kale, banana, mixed berries, Greek yogurt, almond milk, chia seeds, and protein powder (if using) into a blender.

2. Blend on high until smooth and creamy. If the mixture is too thick, you can add more almond milk.

3. Add ice cubes and blend again until the smoothie reaches your desired consistency.

Tips for Weight Loss

Portion Control: While smoothies are nutritious, keep an eye on portion sizes to manage calorie intake.

Balance: Include a mix of fruits, vegetables, protein, and healthy fats to create a balanced smoothie that keeps you full and satisfied.

Choose Unsweetened: Opt for unsweetened yogurt and milk to avoid unnecessary added sugars.

Add Protein: Protein helps keep you full and supports muscle maintenance. Adding plant-based protein powder enhances this aspect.

Fiber-Rich Ingredients: Ingredients like spinach, kale, and chia seeds provide fiber, aiding digestion and promoting a feeling of fullness.

Limit High-Calorie Additions: Be mindful of high-calorie add-ons like nut butter, coconut oil, or excessive fruits.

Hydration: Using water-rich ingredients like cucumber or adding enough liquid ensures proper hydration.

Variation: Change up ingredients to prevent taste fatigue and ensure a broad spectrum of nutrients.

Benefits

- Nutrient-Rich

This smoothie is loaded with vitamins, minerals, and antioxidants from spinach, banana, and cucumber, supporting your overall health and immune system.

- Protein Boost

Greek yogurt and plant-based protein powder provide a protein punch that can help with muscle maintenance and feeling satisfied.

- Weight Loss Aid

The combination of fiber from fruits and vegetables, along with protein and healthy fats, can help control hunger and stabilize blood sugar levels, aiding in weight loss efforts.

This Green Protein Power Smoothie is a great option for those looking to increase their protein intake while still enjoying the benefits of nutrient-rich greens. It's perfect for a post-workout recovery or a filling breakfast option.

Recipe 2

** Green Detox Smoothie**

Ingredients

- 1 cup spinach (leafy greens)
- 1/2 cucumber (peeled and sliced)
- 1/2 green apple (cored and chopped)
- 1/2 banana
- 1/2 cup unsweetened almond milk (you can also use skim milk)
- 1/2 cup water
- Juice of 1/2 lemon
- 1 teaspoon chia seeds
- Ice cubes (optional)

Nutritional Value

This smoothie is low in calories and high in fiber and nutrients. It provides a good balance of vitamins, minerals, and antioxidants from the fruits and vegetables, as well as healthy fats from the chia seeds.

Preparation

1. Combine all the ingredients in a blender.
2. Blend on high until smooth and creamy.
3. If the consistency is too thick, you can add more water or almond milk to achieve your desired texture.
4. Pour into a glass and enjoy!

Tips for Weight Loss

- Use a small banana to control the calorie content.
- Opt for unsweetened almond milk to keep the sugar content low.
- Avoid adding additional sweeteners.

- Focus on portion control. This smoothie is a meal replacement, not an addition to your regular meals.

Benefits

- Rich in Fiber

The combination of spinach, cucumber, and chia seeds provides a good amount of dietary fiber, which can help keep you full and aid digestion.

- Hydrating

Cucumber and the water content of the other ingredients help keep you hydrated, which is essential for weight loss.

- Nutrient-Dense

This smoothie is packed with vitamins, minerals, and antioxidants from fruits and vegetables, supporting your overall health and well-being.

This Green Detox Smoothie is a great way to kick-start your day or to enjoy it as a midday pick-me-up. It's loaded with nutrient-rich ingredients that can help support your body's natural detoxification processes.

Recipe 3

Green Weight Loss Smoothie:

Ingredients

- 1 cup spinach (packed)
- 1/2 cup cucumber (peeled and sliced)
- 1/2 banana
- 1/4 cup Greek yogurt (low-fat)
- 1/2 cup almond milk (unsweetened)
- 1/2 teaspoon grated ginger
- 1 tablespoon chia seeds
- 1 teaspoon honey (optional, for sweetness)
- Ice cubes

Preparation

1. Add spinach, cucumber, banana, Greek yogurt, almond milk, ginger, chia seeds, and honey (if using) to a blender.

2. Blend until smooth and creamy. If the consistency is too thick, you can add more almond milk.
3. Add ice cubes and blend again until the smoothie is chilled.
4. Pour into a glass and enjoy!

Nutritional Value (approx.)

- Calories: 180
- Protein: 7g
- Fiber: 6g
- Healthy fats: 5g
- Vitamins and minerals: High in vitamins A and K, potassium, and magnesium.

Tips for Weight Loss

- Use unsweetened almond milk to reduce calorie intake.

- Opt for low-fat Greek yogurt to keep the protein content high and the fat content lower.
- Limit the use of honey or omit it altogether to reduce added sugars.
- Avoid adding additional high-calorie ingredients like nut butter or sweetened yogurts.

Benefits

- Rich in Nutrients

This smoothie is packed with vitamins, minerals, and antioxidants from spinach, cucumber, and banana, which support overall health and wellness.

- Low in Calories

The combination of low-calorie ingredients makes this smoothie a suitable option for those looking to manage their weight.

- Satiety

The fiber from spinach, cucumber, and chia seeds, along with the protein from Greek yogurt, helps keep you feeling full and satisfied, potentially reducing overeating.

Remember, while smoothies can be a helpful addition to a weight loss plan, they should be balanced with a variety of other nutrient-rich foods and a healthy lifestyle. Always consult a healthcare professional before making significant changes to your diet.

Recipe 4

Green Detox Smoothie Recipe:

Ingredients

- 1 cup spinach
- 1/2 cucumber
- 1 green apple, cored and chopped
- 2 celery stalks
- Juice of 1 lemon
- 1 cup almond milk
- 1 tablespoon chia seeds

Preparation

1. Wash all the fruits and vegetables thoroughly.
2. Place spinach, cucumber, green apple, celery, lemon juice, almond milk, and chia seeds into a blender.
3. Blend on high until smooth and creamy.

4. If the consistency is too thick, you can add more almond milk or water.
5. Pour into a glass and enjoy!

Nutritional Value (approximate)

Calories: ~200
Protein: ~5g
Carbohydrates: ~30g
Dietary Fiber: ~10g
Fat: ~8g

Tips for Weight Loss

- Use water or unsweetened almond milk as the base to reduce calorie intake.
- Be mindful of portion sizes and avoid adding extra sugars or sweeteners.
- Consider using the smoothie as a meal replacement for breakfast or lunch to control overall calorie consumption.

Benefits of the Green Detox Smoothie

- *Rich in Nutrients*

The smoothie is packed with vitamins, minerals, and antioxidants from spinach, apple, and lemon juice, promoting overall health.

- Hydration

Cucumbers and celery are high in water content, helping to keep you hydrated throughout the day.

- Digestive Health

The fiber from spinach, chia seeds, and other ingredients can aid digestion and promote a healthy gut.

Recipe 5

Berry Blast Smoothie

Ingredients

-Mixed Berries
-1 cup Spinach
-1 /4 cup Greek yogurt
-1/2 cup Water

Preparation

To prepare a Berry Blast smoothie, blend mixed berries (strawberries, blueberries, raspberries), spinach, Greek yogurt, and water until smooth.

Nutritional value (approximate for one serving)

- Calories: Around 150-200
- Protein: 8-10g
- Fiber: 4-6g
- Healthy fats: Minimal
- Vitamins and minerals: High in vitamin C, K, and antioxidants

Tips for weight loss

1. Portion control: Stick to recommended serving sizes to manage calorie intake.
2. Use unsweetened Greek yogurt: To avoid unnecessary added sugars.
3. Limit added sweeteners: Opt for natural sweetness from berries and yogurt rather than adding sugar.

Benefits

- Low in calories

The blend of berries, spinach, and yogurt provides a filling, low-calorie option, supporting weight loss efforts.

- High in fiber

The fiber content aids in promoting fullness and regulating digestion, helping you feel satisfied for longer.

- Rich in antioxidants

Berries and spinach are loaded with antioxidants that combat oxidative stress and support overall health.

Recipe 6

** Tropical Paradise**

Ingredients

- 1/2 cup pineapple chunks
- 1/2 cup mango chunks
- 1 ripe banana
- 1 cup kale leaves (stems removed)
- 1/2 cup coconut water
- 1 tablespoon flax seeds

Preparation

To prepare the "Tropical Paradise" smoothie, blend pineapple, mango, banana, kale, coconut water, and flaxseeds in the right proportions according to your taste preference until smooth.

Nutritional Value (approximate)

- Calories: ~250
- Carbohydrates: ~60g
- Protein: ~5g
- Fiber: ~10g
- Healthy fats: ~3g

Tips for Weight Loss

1. Use more vegetables (like kale) than fruits to reduce sugar content.
2. Watch portion sizes and avoid adding extra sweeteners.
3. Include flax seeds for added fiber and healthy fats that can help with satiety.

Benefits of the Tropical Paradise Smoothie

- Nutrient-Rich

Packed with vitamins, minerals, and antioxidants from fruits and vegetables, promoting overall health.

- Hydration Boost

Coconut water helps maintain electrolyte balance and keeps you hydrated, important for weight loss and overall well-being.

- Weight Loss Aid

Low in calories, high in fiber, and with a balanced combination of nutrients, this smoothie can support weight loss efforts by aiding in satiety and controlling cravings.

Recipe 7

****Creamy Avocado Delight****

Ingredients

- 1 ripe avocado
- 1 ripe banana
- Handful of spinach leaves
- 1 cup almond milk
- 1 scoop vanilla protein powder

Preparation

1. Peel and pit the avocado and banana.
2. Place the avocado, banana, spinach, almond milk, and vanilla protein powder in a blender.
3. Blend until smooth and creamy.
4. Adjust the consistency by adding more almond milk if needed.

Nutritional Value (approximate)

- Calories: Around 300-350 calories
- Healthy fats from avocado and almond milk
- Fiber from bananas and spinach
- Protein from protein powder
- Vitamins and minerals from all ingredients

Tips for Weight Loss

1. Watch portion sizes to avoid excess calories.
2. Use unsweetened almond milk to keep the sugar content low.
3. Choose a high-quality protein powder with minimal added sugars.
4. Consider using half a banana if you're looking to reduce sugar intake further.

5. Add ice cubes for a thicker texture without extra calories.

Benefits

- Nutrient-Rich

Packed with vitamins, minerals, and healthy fats from avocado and protein from the powder.

- Satiety

The combination of healthy fats, fiber, and protein helps keep you feeling full and satisfied.

- Weight Loss Aid

Balanced nutrition can support weight loss by providing sustained energy and curbing unhealthy cravings.

Recipe 8

Spinach and Berry Mix

Preparation

1. In a blender, combine a handful of spinach leaves, a cup of mixed berries (such as strawberries, blueberries, and raspberries), half a cup of low-fat milk, a quarter cup of Greek yogurt, and a teaspoon of honey.
2. Blend until smooth and creamy.
3. Adjust the consistency by adding more milk if needed.

Nutritional Value (approximate)

- Calories: Around 150-200 calories
- Protein: 10-15 grams

- Carbohydrates: 25-30 grams
- Fiber: 4-6 grams
- Healthy Fats: 2-4 grams
- Vitamins and Minerals: High in vitamin C, vitamin K, potassium, and antioxidants

Tips for Weight Loss

1. Control Portion Size
   Stick to recommended portion sizes to avoid excess calories.

2. Choose Unsweetened Ingredients Opt for unsweetened Greek yogurt and avoid adding extra sweeteners.

3. Balance Nutrients: Include a source of protein (Greek yogurt), fiber (spinach and berries), and healthy fats (from yogurt) for sustained energy and satiety.

Benefits

- Nutrient-Rich

Packed with vitamins, minerals, and antioxidants from spinach and berries, supporting overall health.

- Weight Loss Aid

Low in calories and high in fiber, aiding in weight loss by promoting feelings of fullness and reducing overeating.

- Muscle Support

The protein from Greek yogurt contributes to muscle maintenance while losing weight, helping to preserve lean body mass.

Recipe 9

Peanut Butter Banana Smoothie

Preparation

To prepare a Peanut Butter Banana smoothie, blend a banana, a spoonful of peanut butter, a handful of oats, a splash of almond milk, a scoop of Greek yogurt, and some ice until smooth. Adjust ingredient proportions to taste.

Nutritional Value (approximate)

- Calories: ~300
- Protein: ~10g
- Carbohydrates: ~40g
- Fat: ~10g
- Fiber: ~5g

Tips for Weight Loss

1. Portion Control: Be mindful of ingredient quantities to control calorie intake.
2. Nutrient Balance: Include lean proteins, healthy fats, and fiber for satiety.
3. Use Natural Peanut Butter: Choose options with minimal added sugars and oils.
4. Choose Unsweetened Almond Milk: Reduces added sugars in your smoothie.
5. Limit Added Sweeteners: Avoid excessive honey or maple syrup.

Benefits

- Satiety

The combination of protein, fiber, and healthy fats can help keep you full and reduce overeating.

- Nutrient-Rich

Offers vitamins, minerals, and antioxidants from bananas, oats, and yogurt.

- Energy Boost

Provides a balanced mix of carbohydrates and healthy fats for sustained energy.

Recipe 10

**Citrus Zing*"

Ingredients

Orange Grapefruit
Carrot
Ginger
Water
Ice

Preparation

To prepare the "Citrus Zing" drink, blend one peeled orange, half a grapefruit (peeled and segmented), one medium-sized carrot (peeled and chopped), a small piece of ginger (peeled and sliced), and a cup of water with ice. Start with these proportions and adjust to taste.

Nutritional value (approximate)

- Calories: 120-150 (depending on size and type of fruit)
- Fiber: 4-5g
- Vitamin C: High content from oranges and grapefruit
- Antioxidants: Abundant from all ingredients, particularly vitamin C and beta-carotene from carrots

Tips for weight loss

1. Limit added sugars: Avoid adding sweeteners to keep the drink low in calories.
2. Hydration: Stay hydrated by consuming this drink as part of your daily fluid intake.
3. Balanced diet: Use this drink as a supplement to a well-rounded diet, focusing on whole foods.

Benefits

- Vitamin C Boost

Oranges and grapefruit provide a high dose of vitamin C, which supports the immune system and skin health.

- Digestive Aid

Ginger aids digestion and can help alleviate bloating or indigestion.

- Hydration and Satiety

The high water content of the drink helps with hydration and can contribute to a feeling of fullness, supporting weight loss efforts.

Recipe 11

** Cinnamon Apple Spice**

Ingredients

- 1 medium-sized apple, diced
- 1/2 teaspoon ground cinnamon
- 1/4 cup oats
- 1/2 cup unsweetened almond milk
- 1/4 cup Greek yogurt
- A pinch of nutmeg (optional)

Preparation

a. In a saucepan, combine diced apple, ground cinnamon, and a splash of water. Cook over medium heat until the apple softens.

b. In a separate bowl, mix oats and almond milk. Microwave for about 2 minutes or until oats are cooked.

c. Once the apple mixture is cooked, combine it with the oatmeal.

d. Allow the mixture to cool slightly, then stir in Greek yogurt.

e. Sprinkle a pinch of nutmeg on top if desired.

Nutritional Value (approximate values)

- Calories: ~300 kcal
- Protein: ~10g
- Carbohydrates: ~50g
- Fiber: ~8g
- Fat: ~7g

Tips for Weight Loss

- Use a moderate portion size to control calorie intake.

- Opt for unsweetened almond milk and plain Greek yogurt to avoid added sugars.

- Focus on portion control and balanced meals throughout the day.

Benefits

- Rich in Fiber

Oats, apple, and Greek yogurt provide a good amount of fiber, which helps you stay full longer and aids in digestion.

- Metabolism Boost

Cinnamon is believed to help regulate blood sugar levels and metabolism, potentially aiding weight loss efforts.

- Nutrient-Rich

This recipe contains vitamins, minerals, and antioxidants from apples, contributing to overall health.

Recipe 12

To prepare a Kale and Pineapple Fusion smoothie, follow these steps:

Ingredients

- 1 cup chopped kale leaves (stems removed)
- 1 cup pineapple chunks (fresh or frozen)
- 1 ripe banana
- 1/2 cup coconut water
- 1 tablespoon chia seeds
- Ice cubes (optional)

Preparation

1. Wash the kale leaves thoroughly and remove the stems.
2. In a blender, combine the kale, pineapple chunks, banana, coconut water, and chia seeds.

3. Blend until smooth and creamy. If desired, add ice cubes for extra chill.
4. Pour into a glass and enjoy!

Nutritional Value (approximate)

- Calories: Around 250-300 calories
- Fiber: 7-9 grams
- Vitamins and minerals: Rich in Vitamin C, Vitamin K, Vitamin A, and manganese
- Healthy fats from chia seeds

Tips for Weight Loss:

1. Portion control: Stick to recommended serving sizes to avoid excess calories.
2. Use fresh ingredients: Whenever possible, use fresh fruits and vegetables for maximum nutrients.

3. Balance: Include this smoothie as part of a balanced diet, combining it with other nutrient-rich foods.

Benefits
 • Nutrient-packed

Kale is a powerhouse of vitamins and minerals, while pineapple provides
Vitamin C and bromelain, an enzyme that aids digestion.

 • Hydration

Coconut water helps keep you hydrated, which can be beneficial for weight loss and overall health.

 • Fiber boost

Chia seeds contribute to the fiber content, promoting a feeling of fullness and aiding in digestion.

Recipe 13

Carrot Cake Recipe

Ingredients

- 1 medium-sized carrot, peeled and chopped
- 1 ripe banana
- 1/2 cup Greek yogurt
- 1/2 cup almond milk (unsweetened)
- 1/4 cup rolled oats
- 1/2 teaspoon cinnamon

Preparation

1. Combine all the ingredients in a blender.
2. Blend until smooth and creamy.
3. If the consistency is too thick, you can add more almond milk.

Nutritional Value (approx.)

- Calories: Around 250-300 calories
- Carbohydrates: 45-50g
- Protein: 10-12g
- Fat: 5-6g
- Fiber: 6-8g

Tips for Weight Loss

- Use unsweetened almond milk to keep the sugar content low.
- Opt for plain Greek yogurt without added sugars.
- Control portion sizes to fit your calorie goals.
- You can adjust the amount of oats based on your carb intake.

Benefits

- Nutrient-rich

Carrots provide beta-carotene, while bananas offer potassium and dietary fiber. Greek yogurt adds protein and probiotics.

- Satiety

The fiber and protein content in this smoothie can help keep you full, aiding in weight management.

- Low-Calorie

With proper portion control, this smoothie can be a satisfying low-calorie option for a meal replacement or snack.

Recipe 14

Blueberry Almond Crunch Smoothie

Ingredients

- 1/2 cup blueberries (fresh or frozen)
- 1/4 cup almonds (unsalted)
- 1 cup spinach (fresh)
- 1 ripe banana
- 1/2 cup almond milk (unsweetened)
- 1/2 cup ice cubes

Preparation

1. Combine all the ingredients in a blender.
2. Blend until the mixture is smooth and creamy.
3. If the consistency is too thick, you can add more almond milk or water.

Nutritional Value (approx.)

- Calories: Around 300-350 calories
- Carbohydrates: 35-40g
- Protein: 8-10g
- Fat: 15-18g
- Fiber: 8-10g

Tips for Weight Loss

- Choose unsweetened almond milk to keep the calorie count lower.
- Stick to reasonable portion size and avoid adding extra sweeteners.
- If you're watching your fat intake, you can reduce the amount of almonds.
- Opt for whole ingredients rather than processed ones.

Benefits

- Antioxidant Boost

Blueberries are rich in antioxidants, which help protect your cells from damage.

- Nutrient Dense

Spinach provides essential vitamins and minerals like vitamin K, vitamin A, and iron, while almonds offer healthy fats and protein.
Satiety

- The fiber from the fruits and spinach, combined with the healthy fats from almonds, can help you feel full and satisfied.

Recipe 15

To prepare a **Mango Ginger Refresher**, follow these steps:

Ingredients

- 1 ripe mango, peeled and diced
- 1 small piece of fresh ginger, peeled and grated
- 1 cup spinach leaves, washed
- 1/2 cup Greek yogurt
- 1/2 cup coconut water

Preparation

1. In a blender, combine the diced mango, grated ginger, spinach leaves, Greek yogurt, and coconut water.
2. Blend on high until the mixture becomes smooth and well combined.

3. If the consistency is too thick, you can add more coconut water to reach your desired thickness.

4. Pour the mixture into glasses and serve immediately.

Nutritional Value (approximate)

- Calories: Around 150-200 calories per serving
- Rich in vitamins (Vitamin C, Vitamin A), minerals, fiber, and probiotics from yogurt

Tips for Weight Loss

1. Watch Portion Sizes: Stick to a reasonable serving size to avoid excessive calorie intake.

2. Choose Low-Fat Yogurt: Opt for low-fat or fat-free Greek yogurt to reduce calorie and fat content.

3. Use Fresh Ingredients: Choose fresh mango, ginger, and spinach for maximum nutritional benefits.

4. Limit Added Sweeteners: Avoid adding extra sugar or sweeteners to keep the drink lower in calories.

5. Stay Consistent: Incorporate this refresher as part of a balanced diet and exercise routine for best results.

Benefits of Mango Ginger Refresher

- Nutrient-Rich

Packed with vitamins, minerals, and antioxidants from mango, spinach, and ginger, this drink supports overall health and immunity.

- Digestive Aid

Ginger can help soothe digestion and reduce bloating, promoting a healthy gut.

- Hydration and Weight Loss Support

Coconut water provides hydration and essential electrolytes, while the combination of ingredients can help you feel full and satisfied, potentially aiding in weight management.

Recipe 16

To prepare **Chocolate Banana Power smoothie**:

1. Gather the following ingredients in the right proportions:
  - 1 ripe banana
    - 1 tablespoon cocoa powder (unsweetened)
    - Handful of spinach leaves (fresh or frozen)
    - 1 tablespoon peanut butter (unsweetened)
  - 1 cup almond milk (unsweetened)

Preparation

2. In a blender, add the banana, cocoa powder, spinach, peanut butter, and almond milk.

3. Blend on high until the mixture is smooth and creamy.

4. Taste and adjust sweetness if necessary, you can add a small amount of honey or a natural sweetener if desired.

Nutritional Value (approximate, can vary based on specific ingredients)

- Calories: Around 250-300
- Carbohydrates: 40-45g
- Protein: 5-7g
- Fat: 10-12g
- Fiber: 7-9g

Tips for weight loss

- Use unsweetened versions of almond milk and cocoa powder to reduce added sugars.

- Limit the amount of peanut butter for calorie control, or opt for lower-calorie nut butter.
- Choose ripe bananas for natural sweetness.
- Ensure portion control and include the smoothie as part of a balanced diet.

Benefits

- Nutrient-rich

The smoothie contains potassium from bananas, antioxidants from cocoa, vitamins and minerals from spinach, and healthy fats from peanut butter, providing a variety of nutrients.

- Satiety

The combination of protein, fiber, and healthy fats helps keep you full and satisfied, potentially reducing your overall calorie intake.

- Energy Boost

The natural sugars from bananas and the combination of ingredients can provide a quick and sustained energy boost, making it a good pre- or post-workout option.

Recipe 17

Peachy Green smoothie

To prepare the Peachy Green smoothie, blend peach, spinach, cucumber, Greek yogurt, and water in the right proportions until smooth.

 The nutritional value will vary based on the specific quantities used, but this smoothie is generally low in calories and high in vitamins and fiber.

Tips for weight loss

1. Focus on portion control to avoid excess calories.

2. Use non-fat Greek yogurt for a creamy texture without added fat.

3. Limit added sweeteners to maintain the natural sweetness of the fruits.

4. Use more vegetables like spinach and cucumber for added volume and nutrients.

5. Experiment with adding ice cubes for a refreshing and filling texture.

Three **benefits** of Peachy Green smoothie

- Low in calories

The combination of peaches, spinach, and cucumber provides a satisfying drink that's low in calories, making it suitable for weight loss.

- . Nutrient-rich

Spinach and peaches are rich in vitamins, minerals, and antioxidants,
contributing to overall health.

- Fiber content

The fiber from spinach and cucumber promotes satiety and aids digestion, helping to control appetite and manage weight.

Recipe 18

To prepare **Raspberry Chia Delight**

Ingredients

- 1 cup raspberries
- 2 tablespoons chia seeds
- 1 cup kale (stems removed)
- 1 cup almond milk
- 1 teaspoon honey (optional)

Preparation

1. In a blender, combine raspberries, kale, chia seeds, almond milk, and honey (if using).
2. Blend until smooth and well combined.
3. Pour the mixture into a glass or bowl.

4. Let it sit for about 10-15 minutes to allow the chia seeds to thicken the mixture.
5. Give it a good stir before consuming.

Nutritional Value (approximate)

Calories: ~180
Protein: ~5g
Fiber: ~10g
Healthy Fats: ~9g
Vitamins and Minerals from raspberries and kale

Tips for Weight Loss

1. Use unsweetened almond milk to reduce added sugars.
2. Opt for a smaller portion size to control calorie intake.

3. Limit or omit honey if you're watching your sugar intake.

Benefits

- High Fiber Content

Chia seeds and raspberries are rich in fiber, which can help promote feelings of fullness and aid in weight loss by reducing overeating.

- Nutrient Dense

Kale and raspberries are packed with vitamins, minerals, and antioxidants that support overall health.

- Omega-3 Fatty Acids

Chia seeds are a source of omega-3 fatty acids, which can contribute to reducing inflammation and improving heart health.

Recipe 19

To prepare the Beetroot Berry Boost smoothie, follow these steps

Preparation

1. Peel and chop a small beetroot.
2. Add a handful of mixed berries (such as blueberries, strawberries, and raspberries).
3. Include a handful of spinach leaves.
4. Pour in a cup of low-fat milk (or a dairy-free alternative).
5. Add a tablespoon of flaxseeds.
6. Blend all the ingredients until smooth.

Nutritional value (approximate)

- Calories: Around 150-200 calories
- Carbohydrates: 25-30g
- Protein: 8-10g
- Fiber: 6-8g
- Healthy fats: 3-5g

Tips for weight loss

1. Control portion sizes to avoid excess calorie intake.
2. Choose unsweetened low-fat milk or milk alternatives.
3. Monitor the number of flaxseeds, as they're calorie-dense.
4. Limit additional sweeteners, such as honey or sugar.
5. Combine with a balanced diet and regular exercise for best results.

Benefits

- Rich in antioxidants:

The mix of berries and spinach provides a good dose of antioxidants, which may aid in reducing oxidative stress and inflammation.

- Fiber content

The blend of ingredients offers a good amount of dietary fiber, promoting satiety and aiding in digestive health.

- Nutrient Diversity

The smoothie is packed with vitamins, minerals, and phytonutrients from various sources, contributing to overall health and wellness.

Recipe 20

To prepare the **Pumpkin Pie Smoothie**, here's what you can do

Preparation

1. Combine 1/2 cup of pumpkin puree.
2. Add 1 ripe banana.
3. Include 1/4 cup of oats.
4. Pour in 1 cup of unsweetened almond milk.
5. Add 1/4 cup of Greek yogurt.
6. Sprinkle in a pinch of pumpkin spice (cinnamon, nutmeg, ginger, and cloves).

Blend all the ingredients until smooth and creamy.

Nutritional value (approximate)

- Calories: Around 250-300 calories
- Carbohydrates: 45-50g
- Protein: 10-12g
- Fiber: 8-10g
- Healthy fats: 5-7g

Tips for weight loss

1. Use a ripe banana for natural sweetness and skip added sugars.
2. Opt for unsweetened almond milk to control calorie intake.
3. Be mindful of portion sizes, especially if using calorie-dense ingredients like oats and yogurt.

Benefits

- Rich in fiber

The oats, pumpkin, and banana contribute to a high fiber content, helping you feel full and satisfied.

- Nutrient-packed

Pumpkin is a good source of vitamins A and C, while Greek yogurt adds protein and probiotics.

- Satisfies cravings

The pumpkin spice provides warm, comforting flavors reminiscent of pumpkin pie, which can satisfy dessert cravings more healthily.

Recipe 21

Minty Watermelon Cooler Recipe

Ingredients (for one serving)

- 1 cup watermelon cubes
- 6-8 fresh mint leaves
- 1/4 cup cucumber slices
- Juice of 1 lime
- 1/2 cup water (adjust as needed)

Preparation

Minty Watermelon Cooler Recipe:
Ingredients (for one serving):
- 1 cup watermelon cubes
- 6-8 fresh mint leaves
- 1/4 cup cucumber slices

- Juice of 1 lime
- 1/2 cup water (adjust as needed)

Preparation

1. Combine watermelon, mint leaves, cucumber slices, and lime juice in a blender.
2. Blend until smooth, adding water gradually to achieve your desired consistency.
3. Taste and adjust lime juice or mint leaves according to your preference.
4. Pour the mixture into a glass, add ice if desired, and garnish with a mint sprig.
5. Stir well before drinking.

.

Nutritional Value (approximate)

Calories: ~45
Carbohydrates: ~11g
Fiber: ~1g
Vitamin C: ~25% of daily value

Tips for Weight Loss

1. Stay hydrated: Watermelon and cucumber have high water content, helping you stay full and hydrated.
2. Control portions: While this drink is low in calories, be mindful of overall calorie intake.
3. Balanced diet: Incorporate this drink as part of a balanced diet, rich in whole foods.

Benefits

- Hydration

Watermelon and cucumber's high water content aids in maintaining hydration levels, essential for weight loss and overall health.

- Low in calories

With minimal calories, this drink can satisfy your sweet cravings without sabotaging your weight loss efforts.

- Nutrient-rich

Watermelon provides vitamins A and C, while mint supports digestion and adds a refreshing flavor.

Recipe 22

Cherry Vanilla Dream Smoothie Recipe

Ingredients (for one serving)

- 1 cup cherries (pitted)
- 1 scoop vanilla protein powder
- 1 cup spinach leaves
- 1 cup unsweetened almond milk

Preparation

1. Place the cherries, vanilla protein powder, spinach, and almond milk in a blender.
2. Blend on high until the mixture is smooth and creamy.
3. Adjust the consistency by adding more almond milk if needed.

4. Pour into a glass and enjoy!

Nutritional Value (approximate)

- Calories: ~250
- Protein: ~25g
- Carbohydrates: ~30g
- Fat: ~5g
- Fiber: ~5g

Tips for Weight Loss

1. Portion Control: Stick to the serving size to control calorie intake.
2. Balanced Ingredients: The mix of protein, fiber, and healthy fats helps keep you full and satisfied.
3. Avoid Adding Sugar: Skip adding extra sweeteners to keep the smoothie low in added sugars.

Benefits of Cherry Vanilla Dream Smoothie

- Protein Boost

The protein powder aids in muscle recovery and supports weight loss by increasing satiety.

- Nutrient-Rich

Spinach adds essential vitamins, minerals, and fiber to support overall health.

- Antioxidant Power

 Cherries contain antioxidants that may help reduce inflammation and support recovery.

Recipe 23

Mango Coconut Bliss

Ingredients (for one serving)

- 1 ripe mango
- 1/2 cup coconut milk
- 1 cup kale leaves (stems removed)
- 1 tablespoon chia seeds
- Ice cubes (optional)

Preparation

1. Peel and dice the ripe mango.
2. In a blender, combine the diced mango, coconut milk, kale leaves, and chia seeds.
3. Blend until you achieve a smooth consistency. If you prefer a colder smoothie, you can add ice cubes.
4. Pour the smoothie into a glass and enjoy!

Nutritional Value (approximate values)

- Calories: ~300 kcal
- Carbohydrates: ~40g
- Protein: ~5g
- Fat: ~14g
- Fiber: ~10g

Tips for Weight Loss

1. Watch portion sizes: Stick to a single serving size to control calorie intake.
2. Balance ingredients: While the natural sugars in mango provide flavor, balance them with fiber-rich kale and chia seeds for satiety.
3. Limit added sweeteners: Avoid adding additional sweeteners to keep the smoothie's overall calorie content in check.

Benefits

- Nutrient-Rich

This smoothie offers a variety of nutrients, including vitamins (A, C, K), minerals (potassium, magnesium), antioxidants, and dietary fiber.

- Weight Loss Support

The fiber and healthy fats from coconut milk and chia seeds can promote a feeling of fullness, aiding weight loss efforts.

- Hydration and Refreshment

The high water content in mango and coconut milk, along with the hydrating

properties of kale, helps keep you refreshed
and hydrated.

Recipe 24

Strawberry Rhubarb Delight

Ingredients

- 1 cup strawberries, sliced
- 1 cup rhubarb, chopped
- 1/2 cup Greek yogurt
- 1/2 cup almond milk
- 2 tablespoons honey (adjust to taste)

Preparation

1. In a saucepan, combine the sliced strawberries and chopped rhubarb.
2. Cook the fruit over medium heat until they soften and release their juices, about 5-7 minutes.
3. Remove from heat and let the mixture cool down.

4. Once cooled, blend the fruit mixture until smooth using a blender or food processor.
5. In a bowl, mix the blended fruit with Greek yogurt, almond milk, and honey.
6. Stir until everything is well combined and you have a smooth mixture.
7. Adjust the sweetness with more honey if needed.
8. Serve the Strawberry Rhubarb Delight in bowls or glasses and enjoy!

Nutritional Value (approx.)

- Calories: ~150-200
- Protein: ~7-10g
- Carbohydrates: ~25-30g
- Fat: ~3-5g
- Fiber: ~3-4g

Tips for Weight Loss

1. Portion Control: Stick to recommended serving sizes to avoid overeating.
2. Use Low-Fat Dairy: Opt for low-fat Greek yogurt and almond milk to reduce calorie intake.
3. Monitor Sweeteners: Use honey sparingly or consider using natural alternatives like stevia to reduce added sugars.

Benefits

- Nutrient-Rich

This dessert provides vitamins, minerals, and antioxidants from strawberries and rhubarb, supporting overall health.

- Protein Boost

Greek yogurt adds protein, which can help increase feelings of fullness and support muscle maintenance during weight loss.

- Digestive Fiber

The fruit and Greek yogurt contribute to dietary fiber, aiding digestion and promoting a feeling of fullness.

Recipe 25

Blackberry Basil Breeze Smoothie

Ingredients

- 1 cup blackberries
- 4-6 fresh basil leaves
- 1/2 cucumber, peeled and chopped
- 1 cup unsweetened almond milk

Preparation

1. Wash the blackberries, basil leaves, and cucumber.
2. In a blender, combine the blackberries, basil leaves, cucumber, and almond milk.
3. Blend until smooth and creamy.

4. If desired, you can add ice cubes for a colder texture.

Nutritional Value (Approximate)

- Calories: Around 100-120 calories
- Carbohydrates: 15-20g
- Fiber: 5-7g
- Protein: 1-3g
- Healthy Fats: 3-5g

Tips for Weight Loss

1. Use almond milk for a creamy base with fewer calories than regular milk or yogurt.
2. Opt for fresh, whole ingredients to maximize nutrients and minimize added sugars.
3. Watch portion sizes to avoid excessive calorie intake.

Benefits

- Blackberries

Rich in antioxidants, vitamins (C and K), and fiber. They can help with digestion, support immune function, and contribute to healthy skin.

- Basil Leaves

Packed with antioxidants and essential oils. Basil has anti-inflammatory properties and can aid in digestion.

- Cucumber

Low in calories and high in water content, cucumber can help with hydration and

promote a feeling of fullness, which can aid
in weight loss.

Recipe 26

Sweet Potato Pie Smoothie

Ingredients (for 1 serving)

- 1/2 cup cooked sweet potato (cooled)
- 1 small ripe banana
- 1/2 teaspoon ground cinnamon
- 1/2 cup unsweetened almond milk
- 1/4 cup Greek yogurt (plain, non-fat)
- Ice cubes (optional)

Preparation

1. Peel and dice the cooked sweet potato and let it cool to room temperature.

2. In a blender, combine the diced sweet potato, ripe banana, ground cinnamon, almond milk, and Greek yogurt.
3. Blend until smooth and creamy. If desired, add a few ice cubes and blend again.
4. Pour into a glass and sprinkle a dash of cinnamon on top for garnish.
5. Enjoy your Sweet Potato Pie Smoothie!

Nutritional Value (approximate)

- Calories: around 200-250
- Protein: around 10-12g
- Carbohydrates: around 40-45g
- Fiber: around 5-6g
- Healthy Fats: around 3-4g

Tips for Weight Loss

1. Portion Control: Be mindful of portion sizes to avoid excessive calorie intake.

2. Substitute Ingredients: You can adjust the sweetness by using less banana or adding a natural sweetener like a touch of honey or maple syrup.

3. Balance with Meals: Incorporate the smoothie as part of a balanced diet and not as a meal replacement. Pair it with lean proteins, whole grains, and plenty of vegetables.

4. Choose Unsweetened Varieties: Opt for unsweetened almond milk and Greek yogurt to cut down on added sugars.

5. Stay Active: Combine your healthy eating with regular physical activity to enhance weight loss efforts.

Benefits of Sweet Potato Pie Smoothie

- Rich in Nutrients

Sweet potatoes are packed with vitamins, minerals, and antioxidants like beta-carotene, which support overall health.

- Fiber Content

The fiber from sweet potatoes and bananas can help with digestion and promote a feeling of fullness, aiding in weight management.

- Healthy Carbohydrates

The combination of complex carbohydrates from sweet potatoes and natural sugars from bananas provides sustained energy.

Recipe 27

** Apple Cider Vinegar Refresher**

Ingredients

- 1 medium-sized apple, cored and chopped
- 1 tablespoon apple cider vinegar
- 1 cup fresh spinach leaves
- 1/2 cup water
- Ice cubes

Preparation

1. In a blender, combine the chopped apple, apple cider vinegar, spinach leaves, and water.
2. Blend until smooth.
3. Add ice cubes and blend again until the mixture is chilled and well-mixed.
4. Pour into a glass and enjoy!

Nutritional Value (approximate)

- Calories: 80-100 kcal
- Carbohydrates: 20-25g
- Fiber: 3-4g
- Protein: 1-2g
- Fat: 0.5g

Tips for Weight Loss Effectiveness

1. Portion Control: Stick to recommended portion sizes to avoid excess calorie intake.
2. Balanced Diet: Incorporate the refresher as part of a balanced diet rich in fruits, vegetables, lean proteins, and whole grains.
3. Regular Exercise: Combine this with a regular exercise routine for effective weight loss.

Benefits

- Aids Digestion

Apple cider vinegar can support digestion and may help alleviate bloating and indigestion.

- Hydration

With its water and fruit content, the refresher helps keep you hydrated.

- Nutrient Boost

Spinach and apple provide essential vitamins, minerals, and antioxidants that contribute to overall health.

Recipe 28

** Blueberry Burst smoothie**

Ingredients (for 1 serving)

- 1/2 cup blueberries (fresh or frozen)
- 1 cup fresh spinach leaves
- 1/4 cup Greek yogurt (low-fat or non-fat)
- 1/2 cup almond milk (unsweetened)
- 1 tablespoon fresh lemon juice

Preparation

1. Add blueberries, spinach, Greek yogurt, almond milk, and lemon juice to a blender.
2. Blend on high speed until smooth and creamy.
3. If the consistency is too thick, you can add more almond milk to achieve your desired thickness.
4. Pour into a glass and enjoy!

Nutritional Value (approximate)

- Calories: ~150-180
- Protein: ~10-12g
- Carbohydrates: ~20-25g
- Fat: ~3-5g
- Fiber: ~4-6g

Tips for Weight Loss

1. Watch Portion Sizes: Stick to recommended portion sizes to manage calorie intake.
2. Opt for Unsweetened Ingredients: Use unsweetened almond milk and plain Greek yogurt to avoid added sugars.
3. Include Lean Protein: To increase satiety, you can add a scoop of protein powder or a tablespoon of chia seeds.

Benefits

- Nutrient-Rich

This smoothie is packed with vitamins, minerals, and antioxidants from blueberries and spinach, supporting overall health.

- Low in Calories

With a good balance of nutrients and relatively low-calorie content, it can be a satisfying yet light option for those aiming to lose weight.

- Hydration and Detox

Lemon juice aids in digestion and can help with detoxification, while the high water content in the smoothie contributes to hydration.

Recipe 29

** Creamy Green Tea Matcha smoothie **

Ingredients

- 1 teaspoon matcha powder
- 1 ripe banana
- 1 cup spinach leaves (packed)
- 1 cup unsweetened almond milk
- 1 teaspoon honey (adjust to taste)

Preparation

1. Add the almond milk to the blender first.
2. Add the spinach, followed by the banana.
3. Add the matcha powder and honey.
4. Blend on high until smooth and creamy.
5. Taste and adjust honey if needed.

Nutritional Value (approximate)

- Calories: Around 220
- Protein: About 5g
- Fat: Around 5g
- Carbohydrates: Approximately 40g
- Fiber: About 6g

Tips for Weight Loss

1. Use unsweetened almond milk to keep the calorie count low.
2. Keep an eye on the portion size and avoid adding excessive honey.
3. Consume the smoothie as a meal replacement or snack, not as an addition to your regular meals.

Benefits

- Rich in Antioxidants

Matcha powder is high in antioxidants, particularly catechins, which can help protect your cells from damage and promote overall health.

- Energy Boost

The combination of matcha and banana provides a natural source of energy without the crash that can come from sugary snacks.

- Weight Management

Spinach and matcha can potentially aid in weight loss due to their metabolism-boosting properties and low-calorie content.

Recipe 30

Green Protein Power Smoothie

Ingredients

- 1 cup spinach (fresh or frozen)
- 1/2 banana
- 1/2 cup Greek yogurt (unsweetened)
- 1/2 cup almond milk (unsweetened)
- 1 scoop of protein powder (whey, pea, or plant-based)
- 1 tablespoon chia seeds
- 1/4 cup berries (blueberries, strawberries, or raspberries)
- Ice cubes (as needed)
- Optional: a drizzle of honey for sweetness

Nutritional Value (approximate)

- Calories: Around 250-300 calories
- Protein: 25-30g
- Fiber: 8-10g
- Healthy Fats: 8-10g
- Carbohydrates: 25-30g

Preparation

1. Add the spinach, banana, Greek yogurt, almond milk, protein powder, chia seeds, berries, and ice cubes to a blender.
2. Blend until you achieve a smooth consistency. If the smoothie is too thick, you can add more almond milk to reach your desired texture.
3. Taste and adjust sweetness by adding a drizzle of honey if needed.
4. Pour into a glass and enjoy!

Benefits

- Rich in Nutrients

This smoothie provides a good balance of protein, fiber, healthy fats, and vitamins from spinach and berries, promoting overall health.

- Satiety

The combination of protein, fiber, and healthy fats helps keep you feeling full and satisfied, reducing the chances of overeating later in the day.

- Metabolism Boost

The protein and fiber content can help support a healthy metabolism, aiding in weight loss by promoting the burning of calories.

Chapter 5: Preservation

Freezing smoothie ingredients

1. **Wash and Chop**: Wash and chop your fruits and vegetables before freezing. This makes it easier to blend them later. Remove any pits, cores, or seeds as needed.

2. **Single Servings**: Portion your ingredients into single-serving portions before freezing. This makes it convenient to grab just what you need for one smoothie.

3. **Freeze in Advance**: Spend some time once a week to prepare and freeze your ingredients. This way, you'll always have a variety of options ready to go.

4. **Flash Freeze**: Lay out chopped fruits and veggies on a baking sheet lined with parchment paper. Freeze them individually

before transferring them to a zip-top bag. This prevents them from sticking together in a big clump.

5. **Liquid Ingredients**: Some liquid ingredients like yogurt, milk, or fruit juices can also be pre-measured and frozen in ice cube trays. This reduces the need for measuring and thins out your smoothie as it blends.

6. **Greens and Herbs**: For leafy greens or herbs, blanch them quickly in boiling water, then plunge them into ice water to retain color and nutrients before freezing.

7. **Labeling**: Label your freezer bags with the date and type of ingredients. This ensures you use them within a reasonable timeframe.

8. **Smoothie Kits**: Create "smoothie kits" by combining complementary ingredients in

individual bags. For example, mix frozen berries with spinach and a banana in one bag.

9. **Seal Properly**: Remove as much air as possible from the freezer bags before sealing. This helps prevent freezer burn and maintains the quality of the ingredients.

10. **Experiment**: Don't be afraid to experiment with different combinations of frozen ingredients to keep your smoothies interesting and nutritious.

Remember, while most fruits and vegetables freeze well, some ingredients like citrus fruits might not freeze as smoothly due to their high water content. Enjoy your hassle-free smoothie-making!

Smoothie texture and Consistency

Achieving different textures and consistencies in smoothies depends on the ingredients and techniques you use. For a thin and drinkable smoothie, use a higher ratio of liquid (such as water, milk, or juice) to solid ingredients. To create a thicker and spoonable smoothie bowl, use less liquid and more frozen fruits, vegetables, or yogurt. You can also experiment with adding ingredients like bananas, avocados, nut butter, or oats to adjust the thickness. Blending for a shorter time results in a chunkier texture, while longer blending yields a smoother consistency. Remember to start with small amounts and adjust gradually to reach your desired texture.

Chapter 6:Garnishing and Toppings

Here are some creative ideas for garnishes and toppings that can add a delightful touch to your dishes:

1. **Savory Options**

   - Microgreens or edible flowers for a pop of color and freshness.
   - Crumbled bacon or prosciutto for a savory crunch.
   - Toasted breadcrumbs or panko for added texture.
   - Roasted garlic chips for a flavorful kick.
   - Shaved parmesan or other hard cheeses for richness.

2. **Sweet Options**

- Crushed nuts (almonds, pistachios, walnuts) for a nutty crunch.
- Fresh fruit slices (berries, kiwi, banana) for a burst of sweetness.
- Chocolate shavings or curls for a touch of indulgence.
- Whipped cream or yogurt swirls for creaminess.
- Sprinkles or edible glitter for a fun and whimsical look.

3. Global Flavors

- Sliced avocado and lime wedges for a Mexican twist.
- Chopped scallions and sesame seeds for an Asian flair.
- Za'atar or sumac for Middle Eastern-inspired dishes.
- Chopped olives and feta cheese for a Mediterranean touch.

- Cilantro and jalapeno slices for a Tex-Mex vibe.

4. **Drizzles and Sauces**

- Balsamic reduction for a tangy-sweet drizzle.
- Pesto sauce for a burst of herbal freshness.
- Chili oil or hot honey for a spicy kick.
- Fruit coulis (berry, mango) for a fruity burst of flavor.
- Maple syrup or caramel sauce for a comforting sweetness.

Remember, the key to creative garnishes and toppings is to complement the flavors and textures of the dish while adding an element of visual appeal. Feel free to mix and match different options to create your unique combinations

Chapter 7: incorporating supplements

Incorporating supplements like protein powder, greens powders, or nut butter into your smoothies can enhance their nutritional value. Protein powder can boost protein intake, aiding in muscle recovery and satiety. Greens powders offer added vitamins, minerals, and antioxidants. Nut butter contributes healthy fats and protein for sustained energy. However, remember that whole foods should remain the foundation of your diet, and supplements should complement rather than replace them. Always consult a healthcare professional before making significant dietary changes.

Storage and shelf life

Storage and shelf life are crucial aspects when it comes to smoothies. They refer to how long a smoothie can be kept without spoiling and losing its quality.

Storage involves properly storing the ingredients before making the smoothie and ensuring the final product is stored correctly. Ingredients like fruits, vegetables, and dairy should be refrigerated to maintain freshness. Once blended, a smoothie should be consumed promptly or kept in a sealed container in the fridge to prevent bacterial growth and maintain its taste and nutrients.

Shelf life, on the other hand, pertains to how long a smoothie can be kept without losing its texture, taste, and nutritional value. Factors such as ingredients used, preservatives (if any), and temperature control impact shelf life. Proper storage techniques extend the shelf life of a smoothie, making it convenient to prepare ahead of time.

The importance of storage and shelf life lies in ensuring that the smoothie remains safe to consume and enjoyable. By following proper storage practices, you can minimize waste, save time, and have a nutritious beverage ready whenever you need it. It's a key consideration for both health-conscious individuals and businesses in the food industry, contributing to a healthier lifestyle and reducing food wastage.

Leftover smoothies should be stored properly to maintain their quality. Ideally, store them in an airtight container in the refrigerator. Depending on the ingredients, most smoothies can be kept for up to 24-48 hours. However, separation and flavor changes might occur over time. If separation occurs, a quick shake or stir before consuming can help. If you're looking to extend shelf life, consider freezing your smoothie in ice cube trays and then transferring the cubes to a freezer-safe bag. This can keep the smoothie good for up to 1-3 months. Just remember to thaw and shake/stir well before consuming.

Storage practices in smoothie making

1. **Prep Ingredients**: Wash, peel, and chop fruits and vegetables ahead of time to make blending easier and save time later.

2. **Use Airtight Containers**: Store prepped ingredients in airtight containers to prevent moisture and air from getting in, which can cause the ingredients to spoil faster.

3. Freeze Ingredients: Freeze fruits like berries, mangoes, and bananas in advance. This not only helps maintain freshness but also creates a colder and creamier texture when blended.

4. **Portion Control**: Measure out the ingredients in individual portions before freezing, so you can easily grab what you need for each smoothie.

5. **Label and Date**: If you're freezing ingredients, label the containers with the contents and date to keep track of freshness.

6. **Pre-Blend Packs**: Create pre-blend packs by combining frozen fruits, veggies, and any other add-ins in separate bags. This makes the blending process quicker.

7. **Liquid Separation**: If you're making smoothies in advance, be aware that some

separation might occur. Simply give it a quick shake before consuming.

8. **Refrigeration**: If you make more smoothies than you can drink immediately, store leftovers in the fridge for up to 24 hours in a sealed container.

9. Minimal Air Exposure: When storing leftover smoothies, choose containers that minimize the amount of air in the container to prevent oxidation.

10. **Glass Jars:** Using glass jars instead of plastic containers can help maintain the taste and quality of the smoothie.

11. **Avoid Over-Blending**: If you're blending ingredients for later consumption, avoid over-blending. This can help preserve the nutrients and flavors.

12. **Add-Ins Separately**: If you're planning to add extras like nuts, seeds, or granola, store them separately and add them just before consuming them to maintain their crunchiness.

Remember, the goal is to keep your smoothies fresh, flavorful, and nutrient-rich. Adjust your storage practices based on the specific ingredients you're using and your consumption timeline.

Creating Unique smoothies

Crafting unique smoothies that are both delicious and healthful is an art that combines flavors, textures, and nutritional goodness. Start with a base of ripe, colorful fruits like berries, bananas, or mangoes to infuse natural sweetness and vitamins. Add a handful of nutrient-rich leafy greens such as spinach or kale to boost antioxidants and fiber content.

To enhance the creaminess, opt for a protein-packed Greek yogurt or a splash of almond milk. For an extra punch of health benefits, consider incorporating superfoods like chia seeds, flaxseeds, or spirulina. These elements not only provide a unique texture but also offer essential omega-3 fatty acids and protein.

Don't forget the final touches! A drizzle of raw honey, a sprinkle of cinnamon, or a dash of vanilla extract can elevate the flavor profile. Experiment with unexpected ingredients like avocado for creaminess or beets for a vibrant hue.

Remember, balance is key. Aim for a harmony of flavors while maintaining nutritional integrity. By blending nature's bounty in creative ways, you'll be able to craft smoothies that satisfy the taste buds

and nourish the body, all in one delicious
sip.

Chapter 8: smoothie nutrition

When creating smoothies, it's important to consider various macronutrients, vitamins, minerals, and other nutritional aspects. Here's a brief overview of each:

1. **Macronutrients**

Carbohydrates: These provide energy and are found in fruits, vegetables, and any added sweeteners like honey or maple syrup.

Proteins: Important for muscle repair and growth. Sources include Greek yogurt, milk, nut butter, and protein powders.

Fats: Healthy fats from sources like avocados, nuts, seeds, and coconut milk can provide satiety and energy.

2. Vitamins

Vitamin C: Found in citrus fruits, berries, and greens, it supports the immune system and skin health.

Vitamin A: Present in fruits like mangoes and dark leafy greens, it promotes vision and immune function.

Vitamin K: Leafy greens like kale and spinach contain this, supporting blood clotting and bone health.

3. Minerals

Calcium: Vital for bone health, sources include dairy products, fortified plant-based milks, and leafy greens.

Potassium: Found in bananas and spinach, it helps maintain fluid balance and supports muscle function.

Magnesium: Nuts, seeds, and spinach are good sources, promoting muscle and nerve function.

4. Other Nutritional Topics

Fiber: Ingredients like fruits, vegetables, and whole grains add fiber, aiding digestion and promoting a feeling of fullness.

Antioxidants: Berries, spinach, and other colorful ingredients contain antioxidants that help fight oxidative stress.

Hydration: Liquid base choices like water, coconut water, or milk contribute to overall hydration.

When making smoothies, try to incorporate a variety of ingredients to ensure you're getting a balance of these nutrients. This can include a mix of fruits, vegetables, protein sources, healthy fats, and liquid bases.

Chapter 9 : Common FAQS

15 common questions about smoothie ingredients, preparation, and health considerations, along with their answers:

1. **Can I use frozen fruits in my smoothies?**
Yes, frozen fruits work well in smoothies and can create a thicker texture without the need for ice.

2. **Is it okay to add vegetables to my smoothies?**
Absolutely! Vegetables like spinach, kale, and carrots can add extra nutrients without compromising the flavor.

3. **What's a good liquid base for smoothies?**

Common options include water, milk (dairy or plant-based), yogurt, and fruit juices.

4. **How can I make my smoothie creamier?**
Adding ingredients like Greek yogurt, nut butter, or avocado can help achieve a creamy texture.

5. **Are there any natural sweeteners I can use?**
Yes, options like honey, maple syrup, agave nectar, and ripe bananas can add sweetness without refined sugars.

6. **Can I use ice in my smoothies?**
Yes, ice can help chill and thicken your smoothie, but using frozen fruits might make it unnecessary.

7. **Should I include protein in my smoothie?**

Adding protein sources like Greek yogurt, protein powder, or nuts can make your smoothie more filling and balanced.

8. **Are there any potential allergens to watch out for?**
Be cautious if you or anyone you're serving has allergies to ingredients like nuts, dairy, or certain fruits.

9. **What's the best way to prevent separation in my smoothie?**
Blending ingredients thoroughly and consuming the smoothie soon after preparation can help prevent separation.

10. **Can I use water instead of milk or juice to reduce calories?**
Yes, using water can help reduce calorie content, but using milk or juice provides additional nutrients and flavor.

11. **Is it possible to make a smoothie ahead of time?**

While fresh is best, you can refrigerate smoothies for up to a day or freeze them for longer storage.

12. **Can smoothies help with weight loss?**

Smoothies can be part of a balanced diet, but portion control and mindful ingredient choices are important for weight loss.

13. **What are some good sources of fiber for smoothies?**

Fruits, vegetables, chia seeds, flaxseeds, and oats are excellent sources of dietary fiber to add to your smoothies.

14. **Are there any specific smoothies for post-workout recovery?**

Including protein, carbohydrates, and electrolyte-rich ingredients like bananas and coconut water can aid in recovery.

15. **Can I make a smoothie that supports immune health?**

Yes, you can incorporate ingredients like citrus fruits, berries, yogurt, and ginger, which are known for their immune-boosting properties.

Remember, individual nutritional needs vary, so it's a good idea to tailor your smoothie choices to your specific health goals and dietary requirements.

Conclusion

In the delightful journey we've embarked upon through the world of smoothies for health and weight loss, we've uncovered a treasure trove of flavors, nutrients, and wellness wisdom. From the vibrant greens that invigorate our bodies to the tantalizing spices that ignite our metabolism, each sip has brought us closer to a harmonious balance between nourishment and vitality.

As you close the final chapter of this book, remember that the path to a healthier you is not just about the ingredients you blend but the intention and mindfulness you infuse into every glass. Smoothies aren't just about shedding pounds; they are about embracing a holistic approach to wellness—one that encompasses the physical, mental, and emotional facets of your being.

In a world filled with fads and quick fixes, the power of whole, natural ingredients and the rituals of mindful consumption remain steadfast. Your journey toward health and weight loss is uniquely yours, and the smoothies you create can be your companions along the way.

So, whether you're sipping on a detox elixir, a protein-packed potion, or a fusion of exotic flavors, let each sip be a reminder of your commitment to yourself and your well-being. May these smoothies nourish not only your body but also your spirit, as you embark on a lifelong adventure of balance, transformation, and self-care.

Cheers to a healthier, happier you—one delicious smoothie at a time.

www.ingramcontent.com/pod-product-compliance
Lightning Source LLC
Chambersburg PA
CBHW070941260726
48661CB00003B/1072